Quick and Easy Balance Exercises for Seniors

Disclaimer

The information provided in this book is intended for educational and informational purposes only. It is not a substitute for professional medical advice, diagnosis, or treatment. Always seek the advice of your physician or other qualified healthcare provider before starting any new fitness program or making any changes to an existing one. The author and publisher of this book are not responsible for any injury or health problems that may result from the use of the information in this book.

Instructed by a Certified Personal Trainer

Contents

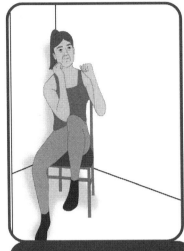

**Elbow To
Opposite Knee**

Pag 09

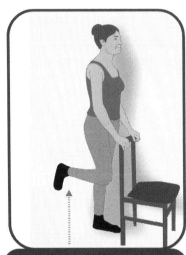

**Chair
Leg Curl**

Pag 11

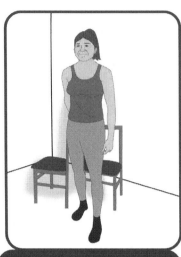

**Stand Up + Step Chair
Assisted**

Pag 13

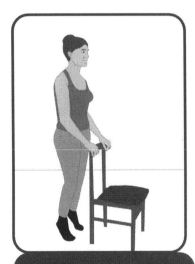

**Assisted
Heel Raise**

Pag 15

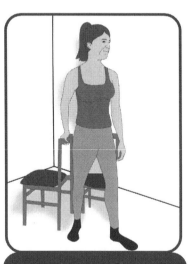

**Stand up + Side Step
Chair Assisted**

Pag 17

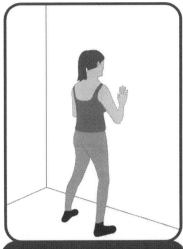

**Assisted
Lateral Stepping**

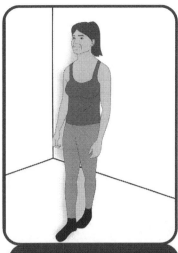

**Tandem
Stance**

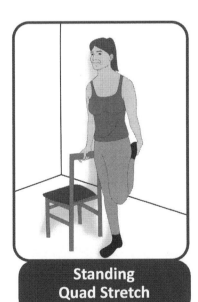

**Standing
Quad Stretch**

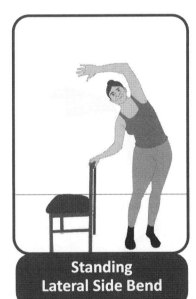

**Standing
Lateral Side Bend**

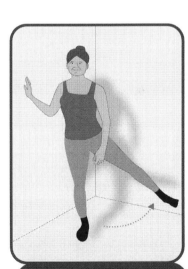

**Abductor Raise
Wall/Chair Assisted**

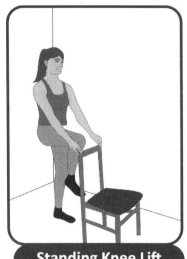

Standing Knee Lift Assisted

Pag 29

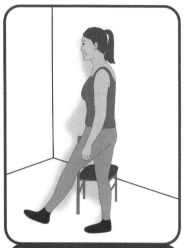

Assisted Two Way Hip Kick

Pag 31

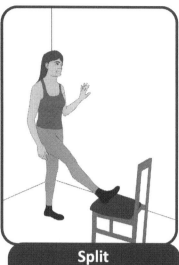

Split Pose Chair

Pag 41

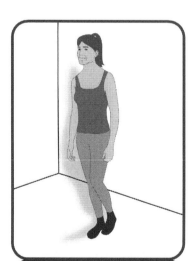

Standing on One Leg

Pag 43

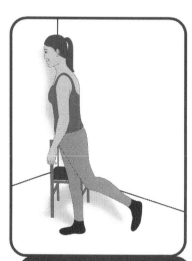

Three Way Hip Kick Assisted

Pag 45

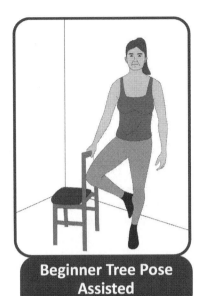

Beginner Tree Pose Assisted

Pag 47

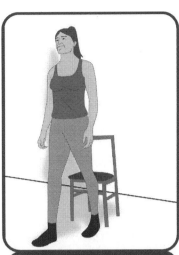

Stand up + Step

Pag 49

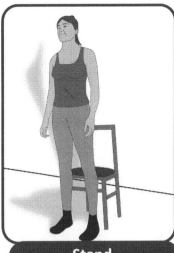

Stand up + Side Step

Pag 51

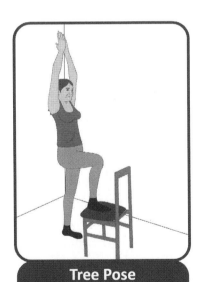

Tree Pose Foot Chair

Pag 53

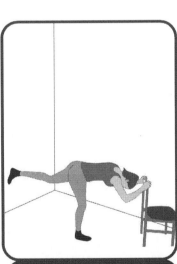

Warrior Pose Hands on Chair

Pag 55

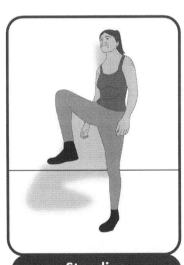

Standing Knee Lift

Pag 57

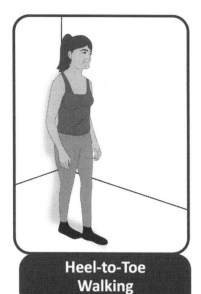

Heel-to-Toe Walking

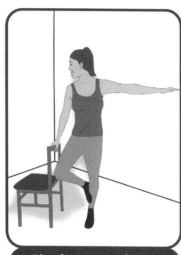

Single Leg T-Shape Chair Assisted

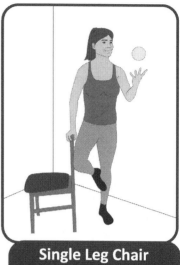

Single Leg Chair Assisted Juggling

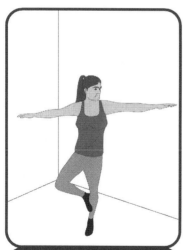

Single Leg T-Shape

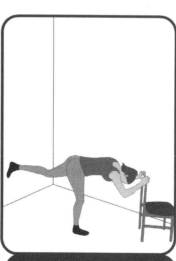

Warrior Pose Hands on Backrest

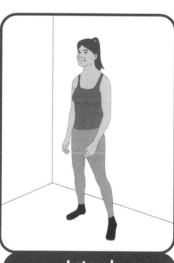

Lateral Stepping

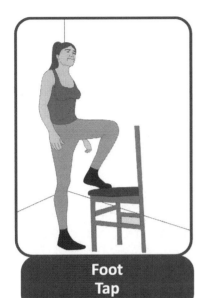

Foot Tap

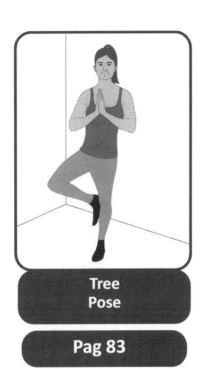

Tree Pose

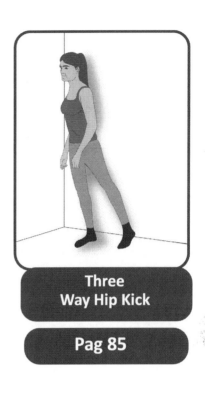

Three Way Hip Kick

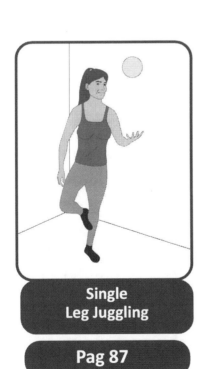

Single Leg Juggling

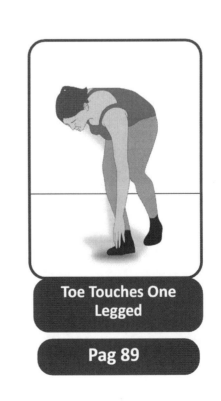

Toe Touches One Legged

INTRODUCTION

Hello there! My name is Alessandro, and I am a Certified Personal Trainer who is passionate about helping people live their best lives by feeling and looking healthier. I love delving into the world of fitness and researching how the human body works to better understand how I can help my clients reach their goals. As a trainer, one of my top priorities is helping people live pain-free, particularly seniors so they can enjoy their golden years to the fullest.

Recently, I came across a shocking statistic that really hit home for me. According to an article I read, falls among adults aged 65 and older resulted in over 36,000 deaths in 2020, making them the leading cause of injury death in that age group. This statistic is staggering and something that I could not believe when I first read it. As a personal trainer, I always knew that my job was to help people become fitter, look better, and move pain-free. However, I never realized the immense impact that falls can have, especially on the senior population. When training seniors, we often focus on balance, mobility, posture and past injuries, but I never fully grasped the importance of fall prevention until I came across this statistic.

It is estimated that 3 million older adults will require emergency room visits due to falls in 2020. This is a concerning statistic, and it really got me thinking about how we, as Personal Trainers, can help. So, I started to dive deep into the topic and researched the best exercises and techniques to help prevent falls among seniors. I learned about the different types of injuries that can result from falls, such as hip fractures, lack of mobility, ankle, and foot surgery, among others. With this knowledge, I felt empowered to help my clients reduce their risk of falling and maintain their independence.

These exercises are taught so that you will improve your posture, become more coordinated and more balanced to move during the day without looking for assistance, regaining confidence in your body!

They will also benefit your mind-body connection as you really have to think how to move and position your body indifferent exercises that you probably have never done before! In fact, on a daily basis you might be struggling now with standing up from the chair or walking without fearing falling down or getting some injuries. Those exercises are designed just for you!

In conclusion, I believe that fall prevention is an important aspect of senior fitness, and I am committed to help you as much as I can with this guide. I am sure you will get amazing results if you perform these exercises for a few weeks!

BALANCE ASSESSMENT: WHERE ARE YOU AT?

This step is not compulsory, and you can skip it. However, it would be interesting to assess your starting level before following the book's guideline.

Here is a 15-20 minute test to assess the balance of seniors, created by Katherine Berg, a well-known physical therapist, more than 30 years ago.

To perform it, you need:

- A six inch step.
- A chair with arms.
- A chair without arms.
- A slipper.
- A stopwatch
- A ruler taped to the wall.

This clinical test is divided into fourteen different steps. These are going to reveal your risk of falling.

Note: Perform these tests next to a person so that he/she can assist you in case you need extra support. Otherwise, do them next to a wall so you can always use it for assistance.

Test 1 - Sit in the chair with no arms, and stand up trying not to use your hands for support (not on your thighs or on the chair to assist you).

Test 2 - Standing for two minutes with feet shoulder width apart without holding onto something (You can use the stopwatch here).
If you can do it, let's skip Step 3.

Test 3 - Sit on the end of the chair with your back straight keeping your arms folded for two minutes.

Test 4 -Stand up and try to sit down without using your arms. Ideally, you would be able to control all the range of motion slowly (very advanced though).

Test 5 - Sitting from the chair with no armrest to the chair with armrest. Ideally you would do it without using your arms (on thighs, armrest or chair) for assistance.

Test 6 - Standing with feet hip width apart with eyes closed for 10''.(Make sure to have someone next to you if you feel that this is challenging).

Test 7 - Standing with feet together for 60''.
Note: if you cannot keep your feet together because your knee gets in the way (they are caving in), try to keep your heels together. If you still cannot, just keep your feet as close as possible to each other.

Test 8 - Stand next to a wall with your arms in contact with it parallel to the floor. Try to reach forward with your arm as far as possible without losing balance. If you have a tape measure how far you can go. Over 10 inches is an amazing result! (Make sure to do both sides.)

Test 9 - Stand up and pick up an object (a slipper works well) from the floor. Have someone next to you in case you need assistance.

Test 10 - Stand and turn all the way around. Then pause and turn around on the other way. Ideally you would do it without the need of holding onto something, and in 4'' or less in total.

Test 11 - Use the step in front of you and take 8 steps on it. Ideally you would do it in less than 20''.

Test 12 and 13- Stand in a stance with your right toes in touch with your left heel, and hold it for 15''. If you cannot do it, put the front foot on the side a bit to make it easier.

If that's still challenging, take a smaller step ahead so that your front foot is not entirely in front of the back foot.

Test 14 - Standing on one leg for at least 10".

Keep track of how you did, and how many tests you could finish with ease, and in which you struggled. I suggest you go back to this test every 4-weeks so that you can assess changes!

HOW TO APPROACH THIS BOOK

If you fear falling, do not feel stable when walking and want to know the best exercises you can do to solve this, this is the right place!

It is key to do some exercises every single day, as it is essential for healthy aging. Most exercises are going to be challenging at first. However, as you exercise daily you will notice great improvements in just a few days!

Also, as you can do these exercises in the comfort of your house, I would highly recommend you to do it barefoot. In fact, this way you are going to work the muscles of your foot that are probably weak right now. By strengthening them, in a few weeks of doing these exercises you will not only increase your balance and live without fear of falling, but also your ankle, foot and knee pain will magically disappear!

The division in three levels allows everyone to start from zero and progress on a daily basis!

BALANCE

There are three main ways in which our body keeps us in equilibrium, preventing falling:

• **Visual**

Have you ever tried closing your eyes and moving, or even standing still? It is way more challenging. Our eyes help us to keep us balanced as they help determine the position of our body in relation to the environment around us.

• **Touch**

The contact of our feet with the floor or any other part of our body with external parts helps improve our awareness and keep us in balance. For seniors, a cane is often used when walking or standing as an extra support. This is due to not only lack of strength but also helps to have more points of contact with the floor.

In this book we are going to focus on exercises that you can do either standing (with support if needed) or sitting. We are going to progress until you reach an elite level of balance for your age, making you feel super confident every time you move, walk, or bend. We do not include lying down exercises as, based on training 1-on-1 dozens of seniors, oftentimes these exercises are quite uncomfortable, so I decided to include only safe and low-impact exercises that provide great benefits in a short time.

Note: There are other ways that help to stay balanced, such as the vestibular way (thanks to our ears and ability to send impulses to our brain understanding our position in the space) but it is not relevant for this guide, and to improve your balance easily and quickly!

To make it easy for you I decided to divide the exercises into three different levels. By training seniors, both in the gym and at -home workout I noticed that you cannot create a training plan as you would in a normal training session. For balance training it works differently.

The best idea is to create exercises designed for each individual that allow seniors to improve step by step.

Beginner exercises are the entry level ones. Those are easy-to-follow safe and low-impacts exercise that you can do seating.

Intermediate exercises are for someone who already has some strength and coordination.

Advanced exercises are what you will accomplish if you follow the guidelines that I am going to provide for you in the next pages.
Lastly, After showing all the exercises, I create a routine just for you to go from Beginner exercises to Advanced ones in just 30 days. This will require 3 days per week of training 5 to 10 minutes.

Note: I encourage you to do some exercises on a daily basis. However, I would not want you to feel the pressure of working out on a daily basis. Hence why I decided to create a plan of just three sessions per week. Obviously, feel free to do each session twice per week!

HOW TO BREATH DURING THE EXERCISES

Breathing is a crucial part of exercise. However, many guides tend to give too many teaching points that make it overwhelming, especially for someone looking for some easy exercises to do at home.

The main tip is to breathe in and out through your nose, if possible, and breathe gently and softly.

A common mistake is to hold your breath. Try not to do that as it would tense your body, and make the exercise more difficult as well as less effective.

BEGINNER EXERCISES

These are a number of easy low-impact exercises suitable for someone who struggles with balance and needs easy exercises to get started.

It is a good idea to stick with these for four weeks before moving on to the Intermediate exercises. This will give you plenty of time to see the results, so that you can set a great foundation for your "balance journey"!

Elbow to Opposite Knee

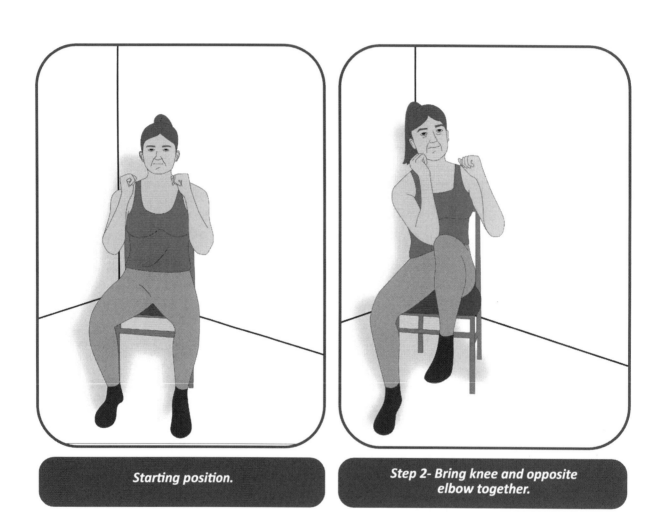

Starting position.

Step 2- Bring knee and opposite elbow together.

How to Do it:

1. Sit on a chair with your back straight and hands next to your shoulders. Elbows bent.
2. Lift your left knee. Bring your right elbow and left knee in contact.
3. Come back into the starting position, and repeat on the other side.

Note:

At first perform this exercise slowly to avoid losing balance. This is very effective as it also includes a semi-rotational movement of your trunk. Great start!

Chair Leg Curl

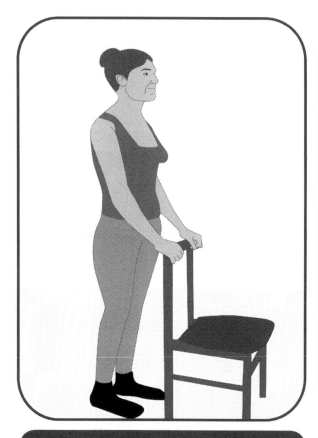

Step 1 – Standing with hands on the chair's backrest

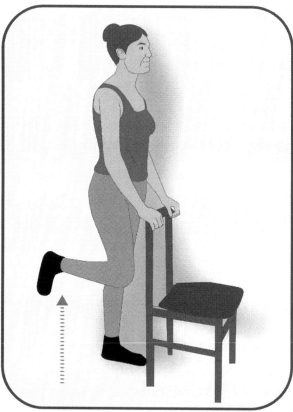

Step 3 – Lifting one leg up with shin parallel to the floor

How to Do it:

1. Put your hands on the backrest of the chair and stand in front of it (a wall works well as an alternative).

2. Bend your knee at 90° and lift one foot up. Hold the position for 1''.

3. After each set, come back down slowly and repeat. Repeat on the other leg.

Note:

Please be very careful (or avoid) this exercise if you feel very weak at your knees. Due to the pressure it places on your standing leg, some people find it uncomfortable.

Stand up + Step Chair Assisted

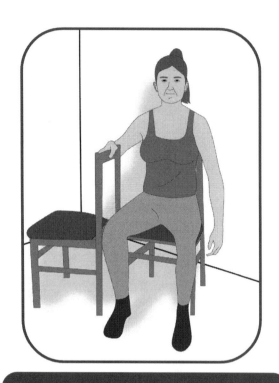

Step 1 - Starting Position

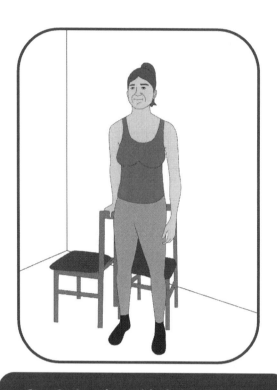

Step 2 - Stand up with chair assistance.

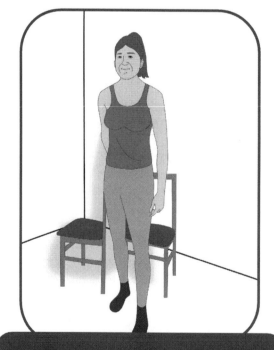

Step 3 - Take a step forward.

How to Do it:

1. Start seating in a chair with another chair next to you to use as a support.

2. Stand up by using one hand on the other chair as assistance.

3. As you stand, take a step forward.

4. Then, sit back again and repeat for the desired amount of reps.

Note:

Remember to switch the leg that performs the step every rep. This is definitely an exercise that has a carryover on daily life activities. In fact, I am sure it happens daily that you sit down and quickly you have to do something, such as answering the phone, opening the door or going to the bathroom. Get better in this exercise, and your life will improve too!

Also, if your chair has an armrest, there is no need to use another chair for support. You can use the armrest to help you stand up.

Assisted Heel Raise

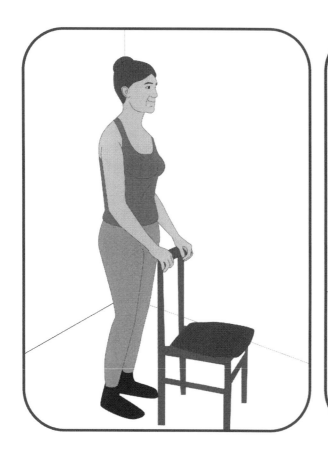 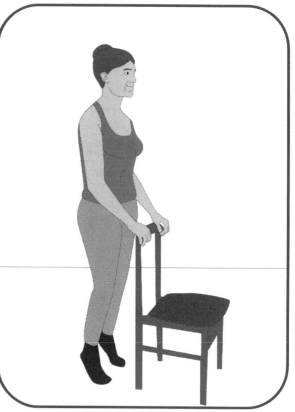

How to Do it:

1. Stand behind a chair's backrest or in front of a wall and put your hands on it.
2. Lift your heels as high as you can and hold that calf contraction for 1''.
3. Come back into the starting position and repeat for the desired sets.

Note:

This exercise is important for your balance as it works your ankle and affects the stability of the foot on the floor. Improving this exercise will help reduce the risk of falling. A great exercise to also avoid ankle injury and aching feet.

Stand up + Side Step
Chair Assisted

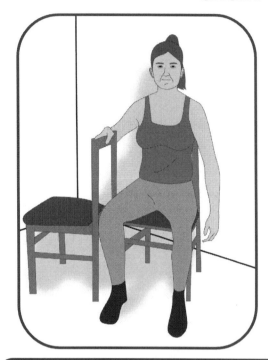

Step 1 - Starting Position

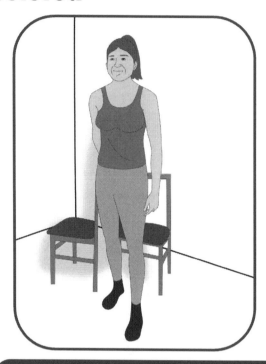

Step 2 - Stand up with chair assistance.

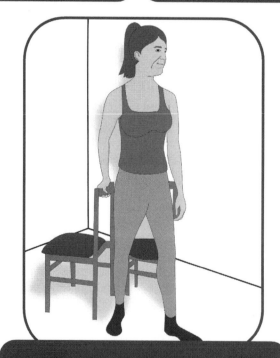

Step 3 - Take a step on the side.

How to Do it:

1. Start seating in a chair with another chair next to you to use as a support.

2. Stand up by using one hand on the other chair as assistance.

3. As you stand, take a step on one side, opening up your hip and body towards left or right.

4. Then, sit back again and repeat in the other direction.

Note:

Very similar to the Stand Up + Step Chair Assisted but with an extra challenge. In fact, this time you are not simply stepping forward but you are stepping to the side. This will require a bit more coordination and hip mobility.

Assisted Lateral Stepping

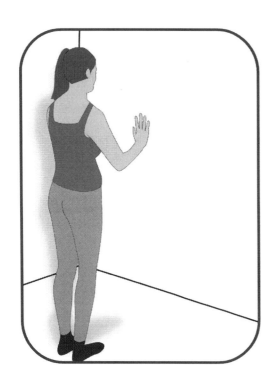
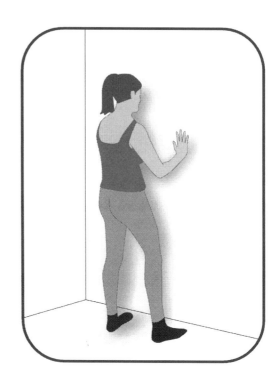
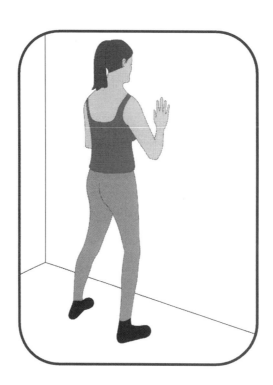

How to Do it:

1. Stand in front of a wall and place your hands on it.
2. Walk with short steps laterally. Your leading foot just goes past your shoulder width in every step.
3. Perform 3 to 5 steps in one direction and then move to the other side.

Note:

A lot of people lose their balance when moving sideways or stepping in tight spaces. This exercise works on it. With the assistance of the wall you can start in a safe and easy way. Give yourself a few weeks and you will be doing this with ease!

Tandem Stance

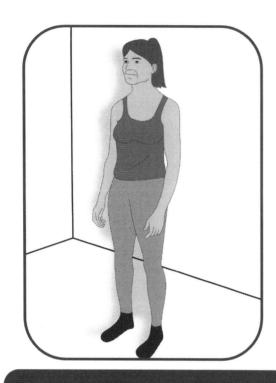

Step 1

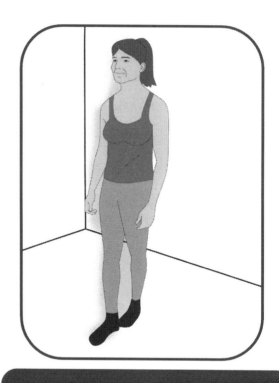

Step 2

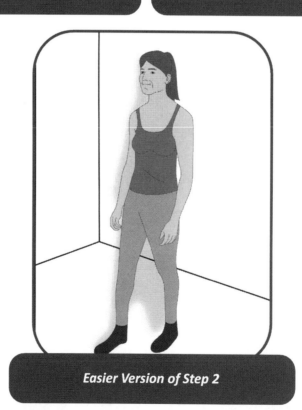

Easier Version of Step 2

How to Do it:

1. Stand tall with shoulders relaxed, hands on your side, and feet slightly closer than hip width apart.
2. From that position, bring your left heel in front of your right toe.
3. Hold this position for 10'' to 20'' (use a chair or wall for assistance if needed).
4. Then repeat switching legs.

Note:

if you do not feel comfortable doing it on your own, do it next to a wall or a chair so you can hold onto something for assistance. As an alternative for making this exercise easier, move your feet apart slightly.

Many people feel shaky once doing it without assistance so it is best to start with something close to you in case you cannot balance anymore. Then, once you feel a bit more confident try spreading your arms. This will help you to feel more balanced. As the weeks go by, you should be able to do it on your own without any problem!

Standing Quad Stretch

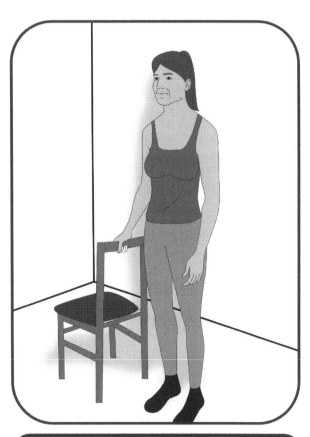

Step 1 - *Starting position next to a chair.*

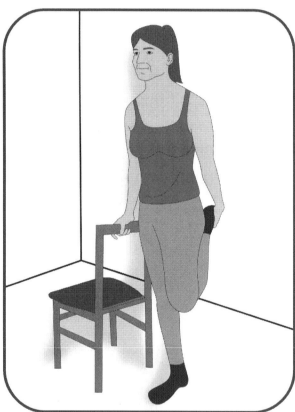

Step 2 - *Final position lifting your left leg and stretching your quads.*

How to Do it:

1. Stand tall with shoulders relaxed, hands on your side, and feet slightly closer than hip width apart.
2. From that position, bring your left heel in front of your right toe.
3. Hold this position for 10'' to 20'' (use a chair or wall for assistance if needed).
4. Then repeat switching legs.

Note:

This exercise is very effective at improving your balance for beginners. Also, it helps prevent muscle tightness. For an extra challenge try not to hold on to the seat.

Standing Lateral Side Bend

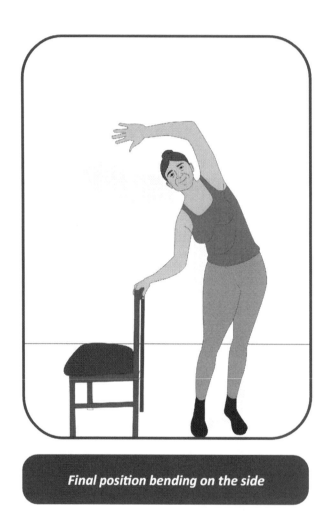

Final position bending on the side

How to Do it:

1. Stand alongside a chair, one-arm distance apart.

2. Place your right hand on the chair's backrest. In the meantime, lift the other arm straight over your head.

3. From there inhale deeply, and then exhale. Once you exhale, bend towards the chair. Stay focused whilst getting into this position.

4. Hold the stretch for 2-5 breaths and then exhale and come into standing pose. Repeat on the other side.

Note:

This exercise, very useful also to stretch the muscles of your trunk, is good to improve balance. In fact, by getting into an unusual position with your body, you will be forced to be extra careful not to fall, making it an amazing entry-level exercise for anyone looking to improve balance and decrease the risk of falling!

Abductor Raise
Wall/Chair Assisted

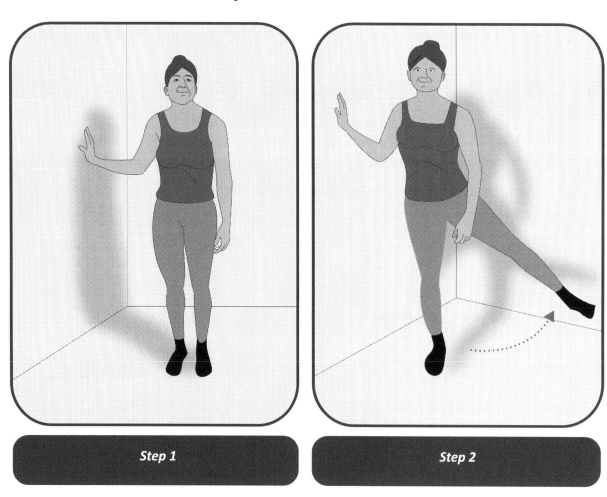

Step 1

Step 2

How to Do it:

1. Stand next to a wall with your right shoulder close to it. Put your right hand in contact with the wall for assistance (you can also use a chair and place your hand on the chair's backrest).

2. Stand on your right leg and lift your left leg on the side as high as you can.

3. Hold that position for a few seconds. Then, come back slowly down into the starting position and repeat for the desired reps.

4. Lastly, Repeat for the other leg.

Note:

Leaning with most of your bodyweight into the wall (or the chair), using it more as a support if you cannot handle all your bodyweight on one leg. Some people, even though it is rare, experience knee pain once they stand on one leg for a few seconds.

Standing Knee Lift Assisted

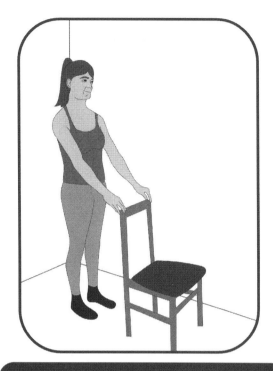

Step 1 - Stand with hands on a chair's backrest.

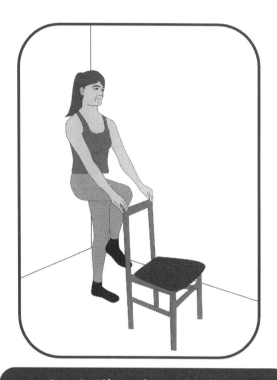

Step 2 - Lift one knee with thigh parallel to floor.

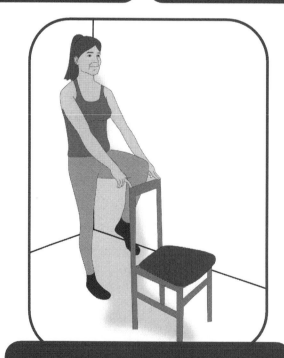

Step 3 -Repeat on the other side.

How to Do it:

1. Stand tall with hands on the side. Have a chair in front of you.
2. Now place your hands on the chair's backrest. This is your starting position.
3. Lift your right leg, bending your knee. Ideally, your thighs will be parallel to the floor.
4. Hold it for 1'', come back slowly down into the starting position. Then, do the other leg.

Note:

At times, when you feel comfortable, try not to touch the chair as a support to make it more challenging and effective!

Assisted Two Way Hip Kick

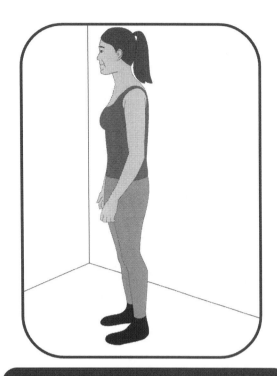

Step 1 - Starting position.

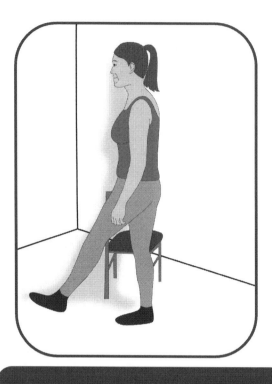

Step 2- ift your leg straight in front of you.

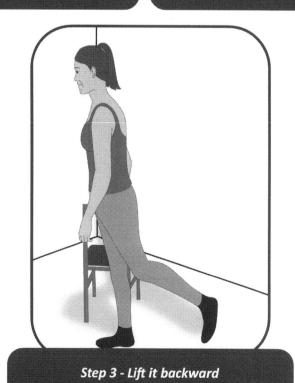

Step 3 - Lift it backward

How to Do it:

1. Stand with your right shoulder next to a chair's backrest and your right hand on it for support. Alternatively, you can use a wall for assistance.

2. Lift slightly your left foot and swing it forward, keeping your leg straight. Hold it for 1''.

3. Come back into starting position, without letting your foot touch the floor, and then move it backward keeping your leg straight. Hold for 1''.

4. Repeat for 5 times and then switch sides.

Note:

This is a great way to start working on your balance with dynamic movements.

4-WEEK WORKOUT BEGINNER PLAN

WEEK 1

DAY 1

EXERCISE	SETS	PAGE
Elbow to Opposite Knee	5 reps for each side	PAG. 9
Chair Leg Curl	10 reps on each leg	PAG. 11
Stand up + Step Chair Assisted	5 reps with each leg	PAG. 13
Assisted Heel Raise	8 reps	PAG. 15
Standing Lateral Side Bend	2 deep breaths for each side	PAG. 25

DAY 2

EXERCISE	SETS	PAGE
Stand up + Side Step Chair Assisted	5 reps with each leg	PAG. 17
Assisted Lateral Stepping	5 steps on each side	PAG. 19
Tandem Stance	10'' each stance	PAG. 21

DAY 3

EXERCISE	SETS	PAGE
Standing Quad Stretch	10'' each side	PAG. 23
Abductor Raise Wall/ Chair Assisted	5 reps for each side	PAG. 27
Standing Knee Lift Assisted	5 reps for each side	PAG. 29
Assisted Two Way Hip Kick	5 reps for each side	PAG. 31

WEEK 2

DAY 1

EXERCISE	SETS	PAGE
Elbow to Opposite Knee	8 reps for each side	PAG. 9
Chair Leg Curl	15 reps on each leg	PAG. 11
Stand up + Step Chair Assisted	8 reps with each leg	PAG. 13
Assisted Heel Raise	10 reps	PAG. 15
Standing Lateral Side Bend	3 deep breaths for each side	PAG. 25

DAY 2

EXERCISE	SETS	PAGE
Stand up + Side Step Chair Assisted	8 reps with each leg	PAG. 17
Assisted Lateral Stepping	6 steps on each side	PAG. 19
Tandem Stance	15'' each stance	PAG. 21

DAY 3

EXERCISE	SETS	PAGE
Standing Quad Stretch	15'' each side	PAG. 23
Abductor Raise Wall/ Chair Assisted	6 reps for each side	PAG. 27
Standing Knee Lift Assisted	7 reps for each side	PAG. 29
Assisted Two Way Hip Kick	5 reps for each side	PAG. 31

WEEK 3

DAY 1

EXERCISE	SETS	PAGE
Elbow to Opposite Knee	10 reps for each side	PAG. 9
Chair Leg Curl	2 sets of 10 reps on each leg	PAG. 11
Stand up + Step Chair Assisted	10 reps with each leg	PAG.13
Assisted Heel Raise	12 reps	PAG. 15
Standing Lateral Side Bend	4 deep breaths for each side	PAG. 25

DAY 2

EXERCISE	SETS	PAGE
Stand up + Side Step Chair Assisted	10 reps with each leg	PAG. 17
Assisted Lateral Stepping	7 steps on each side	PAG. 19
Tandem Stance	15'' each stance	PAG. 21

DAY 3

EXERCISE	SETS	PAGE
Standing Quad Stretch	15" each side	PAG. 23
Abductor Raise Wall/ Chair Assisted	7 reps for each side	PAG. 27
Standing Knee Lift Assisted	9 reps for each side	PAG. 29
Assisted Two Way Hip Kick	5 reps for each side	PAG. 31

WEEK 4

DAY 1

EXERCISE	SETS	PAGE
Elbow to Opposite Knee	12 reps for each side	PAG. 9
Chair Leg Curl	3 sets of 15 reps on each leg	PAG. 11
Stand up + Step Chair Assisted	12 reps with each leg	PAG. 13
Assisted Heel Raise	12 reps	PAG. 15
Standing Lateral Side Bend	5 deep breaths for each side	PAG. 25

DAY 2

EXERCISE	SETS	PAGE
Stand up + Side Step Chair Assisted	12 reps with each leg	PAG. 17
Assisted Lateral Stepping	8 steps on each side	PAG. 19
Tandem Stance	20'' each stance	PAG. 21

DAY 3

EXERCISE	SETS	PAGE
Standing Quad Stretch	15'' each side	PAG. 23
Abductor Raise Wall/ Chair Assisted	8 reps for each side	PAG. 27
Standing Knee Lift Assisted	10 reps for each side	PAG. 29
Assisted Two Way Hip Kick	5 reps for each side	PAG. 31

INTERMEDIATE EXERCISES

Well done, you are making progress! These exercises are slightly more advanced and there will be less assistance when standing on one leg. you will be very confident in your body once you can do all these exercises with ease.

On average, people tend to master these exercises in 5 to 8 weeks. However, following the 4-week Intermediate plan (showed after the intermediate exercises), you will be able to do all of these in just 4 weeks!

Split Pose Chair

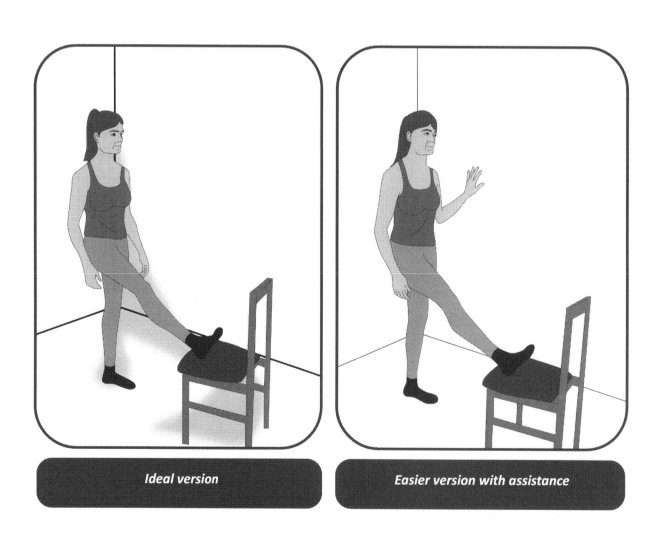

Ideal version

Easier version with assistance

How to Do it:

1. Stand three feet away in front of a chair with shoulders relaxed, and chest up.

2. Place your right heel on the seat keeping your leg straight.

3. Breathe softly in this position for 2 to 3 seconds, and then come back into the starting position.

Note:

This exercise is slightly more advanced than the previous exercises. Now you get the idea of what it means to have all the weight on one leg. It also helps to be able to coordinate your body with unusual movements. If that's too difficult, start with a wall next to you for assistance.

Standing on One Leg

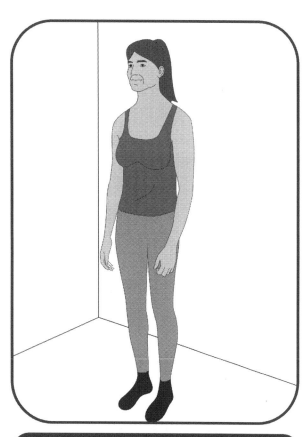

Step 1 - Starting position standing.

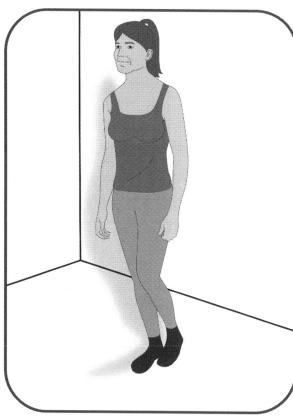

Step 2 - Final position lifting one leg.

How to Do it:

1. Stand tall with feet slightly closer than hip-width apart and chest up.

2. Lift one foot slightly off the floor, and balance yourself only on the other leg.

3. Hold that position for 10-30'' and then repeat on the other side. Hands on the side, or spread them apart for more assistance.

Note:

If you can choose only one exercise to do, perform this one! The benefits are great and will give you confidence when walking. Use a chair next to you if you do not feel safe doing it without any assistance. Instead, if it feels too easy, try closing your eyes whilst doing it. It will be very challenging! As mentioned in the introduction, our eyes help a lot to keep us balanced. Closing them will make every exercise way more difficult.

Three Way Hip Kick Assisted

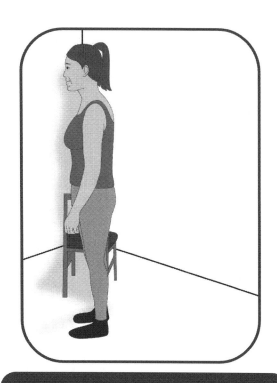

Step 1 - Starting position.

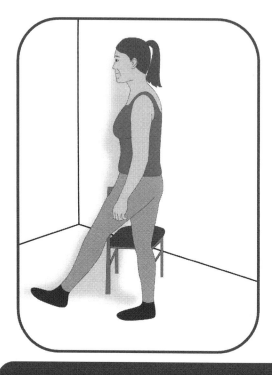

Step 2 - Bring your leg forward.

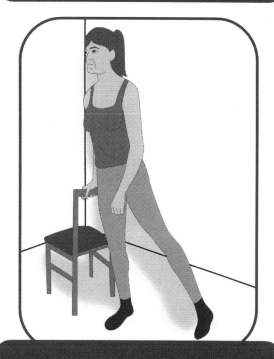

Step 3 - Lift your leg sideways.

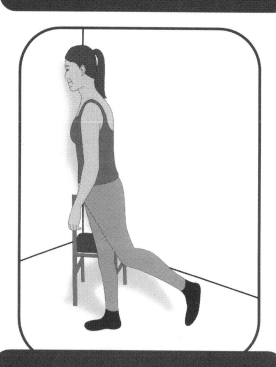

Step 4 - Now lift it backward.

How to Do it:

1. Stand with your right shoulder next to a chair's backrest and your right hand on it for support. Alternatively, you can use a wall for assistance.

2. Lift slightly your left foot and swing it forward, keeping your leg straight. Hold it for 1''.

3. Come back into starting position, without letting your foot touch the floor, and then move it sideways. Hold it for 1''.

4. Once again, come back into starting position and then move it backwards keeping your leg straight. Hold it for 1''.

5. Repeat for 3 to 5 times and then switch sides.

Note:

This is a great way to both work on your balance as well as increasing your hip mobility and strength.

Beginner Tree Pose Assisted

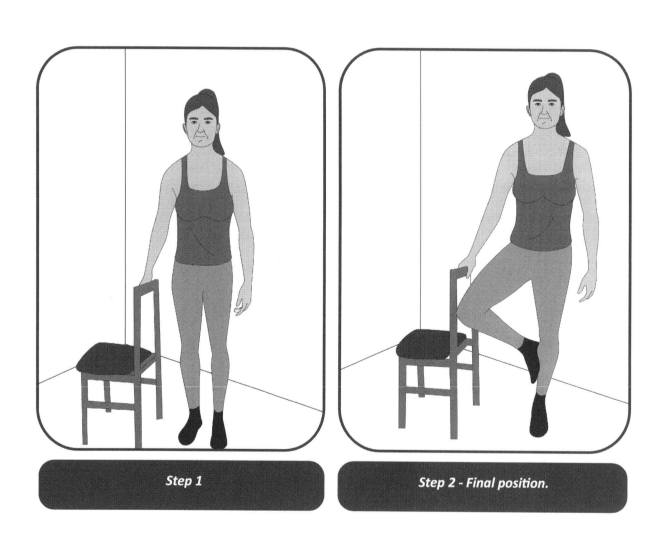

Step 1

Step 2 - Final position.

How to Do it:

1. Stand with your right side next to a chair or wall with your chest up and shoulders down.

2. Place your right hand on the chair's backrest or on the wall for support.

3. Now shift the weight to your left foot lifting the right foot, placing it on the side of your left shin.

4. Hold that position for 10-20'' and then repeat switching sides.

Note:

Feel free to position your foot just below your knee or just above your ankle. As long as all your body is held by only one foot, you are doing it right!

Stand up + Step

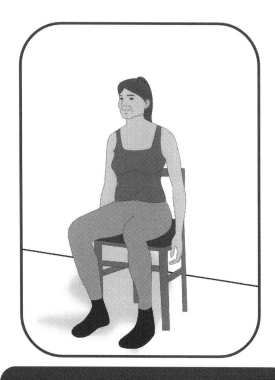

Step 1- Sitting on a chair.

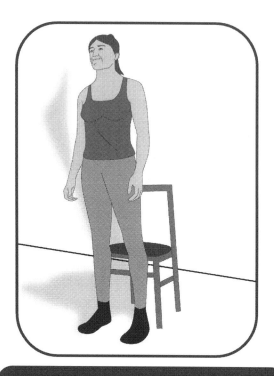

Step 2 - Stand up.

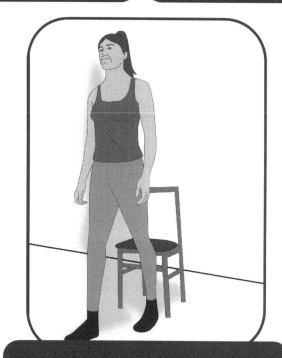

Step 3 - Take a step forward.

How to Do it:

1. Start sitting in a chair with back straight, shoulder relaxed and hands on your thighs.

2. Stand up by only using your feet, without holding onto anything, keeping your hands on your thighs.

3. Then, as soon as you stand, take a step forward.

4. Lastly, come back into the seating position and repeat for 5-10 times.

Note:

Remember to switch the leg that performs the step every rep. This is definitely an exercise that has a carryover on daily life activities. It is a progression of "Stand up + Step Chair Assisted" shown at pag.13.

Stand up + Side Step

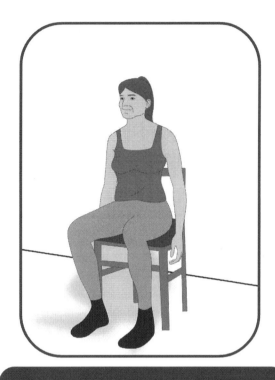

Step 1- Sitting on a chair.

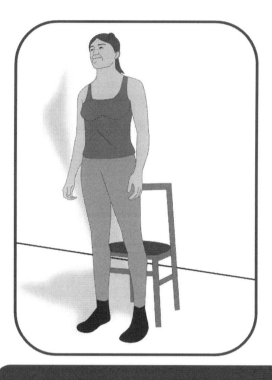

Step 2 - Stand up.

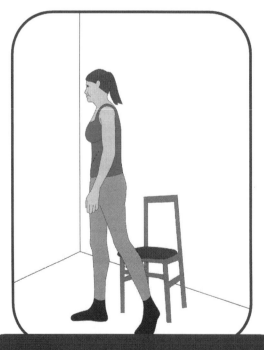

Step 3 - Step on the side.

How to Do it:

1. Start sitting in a chair with your back straight, shoulder relaxed and hands on your thighs.

2. Stand up by only using your feet, without holding onto anything, keeping your hands on your thighs.

3. As you stand, take a step on one side, opening your hips and body towards left or right.

4. Then, sit back again and repeat in the other direction.

Note:

Very similar to the previous exercise but with an extra challenge. In fact, this time you are not simply stepping forward, but you are stepping to the side. This will require a bit more coordination and hip mobility.

Once you can master this as well as the exercise in the previous page, you will feel way better than you used to, having the physical ability and mental confidence to perform daily movements with ease.

Tree Pose Foot Chair

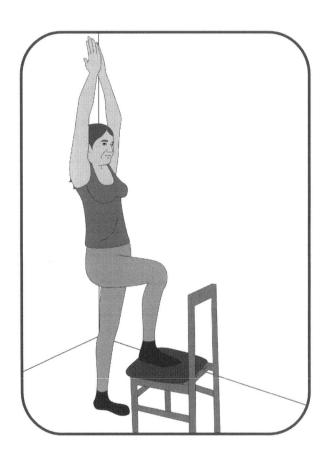

How to Do it:

1. Stand in front of a chair with shoulders relaxed, chest up, and hands on your side.

2. Place your right foot on the chair bending your knees at 90°.

3. Lift your arms over your head. Keep them straight.

4. Breathe softly and deeply 2 to 5 times in this position, and then come back into the starting position.

Note:

Great exercise to get used to staying on one leg, improve coordination and decrease risk of falling.

Walking Backwards Assisted

How to Do it:

Simply find a space in which you can walk for a few steps backward and forward in your house next to a wall for support (or if you have a cane, feel free to use it).

Note: According to research, more than one-third of people over 60 in the US experience injuries from falling every year (Dufek, et al. 2009).

Can you walk forward? If you answered yes, try practicing walking backward, just a few minutes per day. This might seem odd but studies from DeMark and colleagues (2019) showed how practicing this exercise alone for 4 weeks a few minutes per day prevents falling and increases balance in elderly.

Warrior Pose Hands on Chair

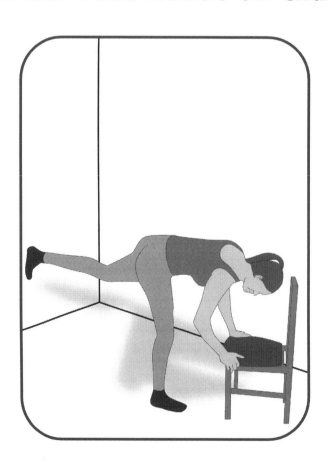

How to Do it:

1. Stand in front of the seat of a chair two feet away from it.

2. From this position, straighten your arms and lean forward so that your hands are on the seat of the chair.

3. Once you do this, lift your leg backwards, keeping it straight. Ideally you would have it parallel to the floor.

4. Hold that position for a few seconds, then rest your leg back to the floor and, whilst still having your hands on the chair, switch legs.

Note:

If you feel discomfort on your low back if you do this, use the backseat of the chair so that you do not have to lean forwards and use your low back excessively.

Standing Knee Lift

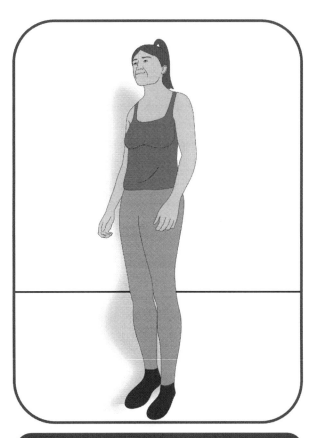

Step 1 - Starting position.

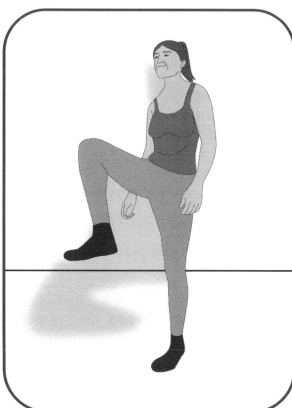

Step 2- Final position lifting your thigh.

How to Do it:

1. Stand tall with hands on the side and feet hip-width apart.

2. Lift your right leg, bending your knee. Ideally, your thigh will be parallel to the floor.

3. Hold it for 1'', come back slowly down into the starting position, do it for 5 to 10 times. Then perform the same movement with the left leg.

Note:

For an extra challenge, when comfortable doing it for reps, try closing your eyes when performing the exercise.

Heel-to-Toe Walking

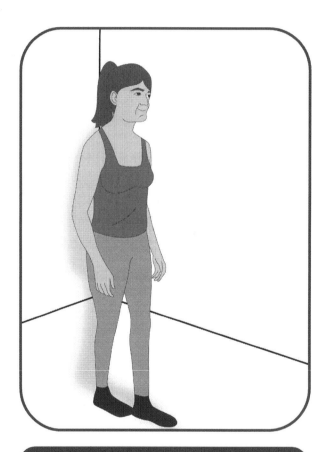

Take steps placing your toes against your heel,
and keep moving forward

How to Do it:

1. Before starting, make sure to have some space in front of you.

2. Stand tall and start walking, placing your right foot heel in contact with your left foot toe.

3. Then, place your left heel against the right toe and keep walking.

Note:

Imagine there's an imaginary line that you are walking on.

Spread your arms for extra balance (or use a cane or a wall for extra support). Instead, for an extra challenge in case that's too easy, close your eyes whilst walking.

Single Leg T-Shape
Chair Assisted

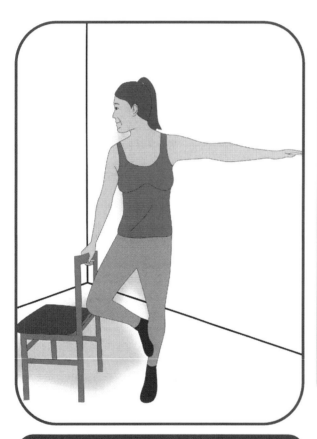

Step 1 - Looking on one side

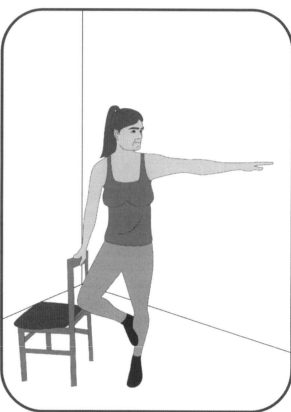

Step 2- Looking on the opposite side mantainning balance on one leg (with assistance).

How to Do it:

1. Stand on your left leg and open the left arm parallel to the floor. The right arm is in contact with a chair for assistance.

2. From there, simply move the head side to side in a slow and controlled manner.

3. Repeat for 5-8 times on each side and then switch legs.

Note:

As you progress, try using the chair less and less for support. Once you feel like you can do it even without a chair, jump at page 75 to do "Single Leg T-Shape".

Single Leg Chair Assisted Juggling

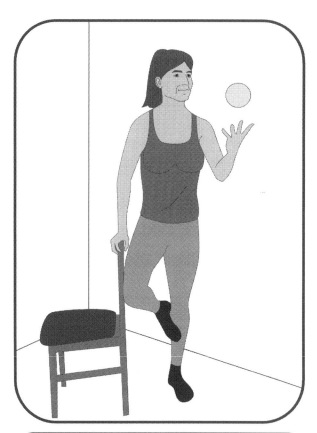

Step 1 - Throw the ball in the air and catch it standing on one leg (with chair assistance).

How to Do it:

1. Stand on your left leg with a chair on your right side.
2. Grab a small size ball with your left hand and place your right hand on the chair's backrest for assistance.
3. From there, throw the ball a few inches in the air and grab it again, still balancing on the left foot.
4. Do it for 10-20 times and the switch side.

Note:

This exercise is going to be fun! Plenty of people did it before and they found it very entertaining. Just 1-2 minutes of this a few times per week will be enough to see amazing results and improvements.

4-WEEK WORKOUT INTERMEDIATE PLAN

Bonus: Walking Backwards Assisted (pag.55) , perform 5 to 10 minutes on a daily basis. This can be done in the comfort of your home, or outside.

You can perform this either before or after the workout, or in another moment of the day.

Based on the amount of time you have and the energy level, you might perform these exercises for more sets.

For example, Day 1 includes four exercises. The minimum would be to do these four exercises, and end the workout there. However, you can perform it one or two more times.

It means that after having completed "Heel-to-Toe Walking" You will do them all over again, once or twice more.

WEEK 1

DAY 1 - Perform 1 to 3 sets.

EXERCISE	SETS	PAGE
Split Pose Chair	3 reps on each leg, alternating	PAG. 41
Beginner Tree Pose Assisted	10'' for each side	PAG. 47
Tree Pose Foot Chair	2 deep breaths for each side	PAG. 53
Heel to Toe Walking	10 steps	PAG. 59

DAY 2 - Perform 1 to 3 sets.

EXERCISE	SETS	PAGE
Standing on One Leg	2 reps of 10'' each side	PAG. 43
Stand up + Step	5 reps for each side, alternating stepping foot	PAG. 49
Warrior Pose Hands on Chair	3 reps for each side	PAG. 55
Single Leg T Shape Chair Assisted	5 times for each leg	PAG. 61

DAY 3 - Perform 1 to 3 sets.

EXERCISE	SETS	PAGE
Standing on One Leg	2 reps of 10'' each side	PAG. 43
Three Way Hip Kick Assisted	3 reps on each side	PAG. 45
Stand up + Side Step	5 reps for each side, alternating	PAG. 51
Standing Knee Lift	5 reps for each leg	PAG. 57
Single Leg Chair Assisted Juggling	10 throws for each leg	PAG. 63

WEEK 2

DAY 1 - Perform 1 to 3 sets.

EXERCISE	SETS	PAGE
Split Pose Chair	4 reps on each leg, alternating	PAG. 41
Beginner Tree Pose Assisted	15" for each side	PAG. 47
Tree Pose Foot Chair	3 deep breaths for each side	PAG. 53
Heel to Toe Walking	12 steps	PAG. 59

DAY 2 - Perform 1 to 3 sets.

EXERCISE	SETS	PAGE
Standing on One Leg	2 reps of 15" each side	PAG. 43
Stand up + Step	6 reps for each side, alternating stepping foot	PAG. 49
Warrior Pose Hands on Chair	3 reps for each side	PAG. 55
Single Leg T Shape Chair Assisted	6 times for each leg	PAG. 61

DAY 3 - Perform 1 to 3 sets.

EXERCISE	SETS	PAGE
Standing on One Leg	2 reps of 15'' each side	PAG. 43
Three Way Hip Kick Assisted	4 reps on each side	PAG. 45
Stand up + Side Step	6 reps for each side, alternating	PAG. 51
Standing Knee Lift	7 reps for each leg	PAG. 57
Single Leg Chair Assisted Juggling	15 throws for each leg	PAG. 63

WEEK 3

DAY 1 - Perform 2 to 4 sets.

EXERCISE	SETS	PAGE
Split Pose Chair	5 reps on each leg, alternating	PAG. 41
Beginner Tree Pose Assisted	20'' for each side	PAG. 47
Tree Pose Foot Chair	4 deep breaths for each side	PAG. 53
Heel to Toe Waking	14 steps	PAG. 59

DAY 2 - Repeat 2 to 4 times

EXERCISE	SETS	PAGE
Standing on One Leg	2 reps of 20'' each side	PAG. 43
Stand up + Step	7 reps for each side, alternating stepping foot	PAG. 49
Warrior Pose Hands on Chair	4 reps for each side	PAG. 55
Single Leg T Shape Chair Assisted	7 times	PAG. 61

DAY 3 - Perform 2 to 4 sets.

EXERCISE	SETS	PAGE
Standing on One Leg	2 reps of 20'' each side	PAG. 43
Three Way Hip Kick Assisted	4 reps on each side	PAG. 45
Stand up + Side Step	7 reps for each side, alternating	PAG. 51
Standing Knee Lift	9 reps for each leg	PAG. 57
Single Leg Chair Assisted Juggling	15 throws for each leg	PAG. 63

WEEK 4

DAY 1 - Perform 2 to 4 sets.

EXERCISE	SETS	PAGE
Split Pose Chair	5 reps on each leg, alternating	PAG. 41
Beginner Tree Pose Assisted	2 sets of 20'' for each side	PAG. 47
Tree Pose Foot Chair	5 deep breaths for each side	PAG. 53
Heel to Toe Walking	16 steps	PAG. 59

DAY 2 - Perform 2 to 4 sets.

EXERCISE	SETS	PAGE
Standing on One Leg	2 reps of 25'' each side	PAG. 43
Stand up + Step	8 reps for each side, alternating stepping foot	PAG. 49
Warrior Pose Hands on Chair	5 reps for each side	PAG. 55
Single Leg T Shape Chair Assisted	8 times	PAG. 61

DAY 3 - Perform 2 to 4 sets.

EXERCISE	SETS	PAGE
Standing on One Leg	1 reps of 30'' each side	PAG. 43
Three Way Hip Kick Assisted	5 reps on each side	PAG. 45
Stand up + Side Step	8 reps for each side, alternating	PAG. 51
Standing Knee Lift	10 reps for each leg	PAG. 57
Single Leg Chair Assisted Juggling	20 throws for each leg	PAG. 63

ADVANCED EXERCISES

Welcome to the elite!

These exercises are very advanced. If you master Intermediate exercises, it might still require some time before you master these. However, once you can master Single Leg Juggling at pag.87 and Toe Touches One-Legged at pag.89 you will avoid the risk of falling forever, improve the ability to move independently, and overall feel like in your prime years.

You might want to perform exercises at least 3x per week with sessions of 5-10 min per day.

However, feel free to repeat those sessions twice per week for a total of 6 times per week.

For example:

WEEK 1

Monday - Day 1

Tuesday - Day 2

Wednesday - Day 3

Thursday - Day 1

Friday - Day 2

Saturday - Day 3

Sunday - Rest

Single Leg T-Shape

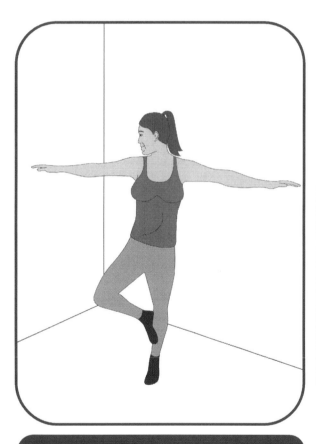

Step 1 -Starting position.

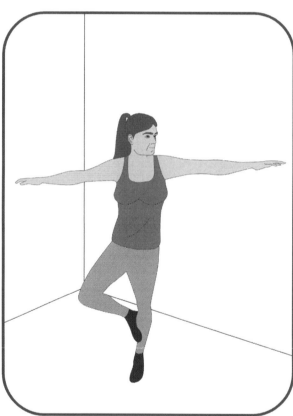

Then , look on the other side.

How to Do it:

1. Stand on your left leg and open the arms parallel to the floor. The right foot is not touching the floor.

2. From there, simply move the head side to side looking first at your right hand, and then at your left hand.

3. Repeat for 5-10 times on each side and then switch legs.

Note:

Very challenging exercise...But if you made it this far, I am sure you got this! Start with just a few reps on each side and build up slowly. This exercise is the progression of "Single Leg T-Shape Chair Assisted" at page 61.

Warrior Pose Hands on Backrest

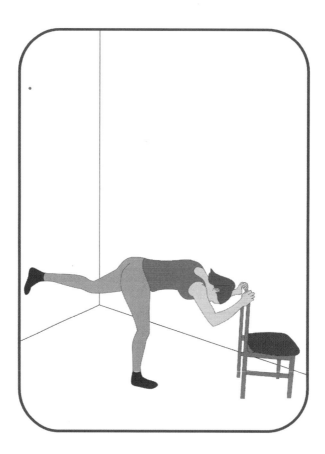

How to Do it:

1. Stand in front of the seat of a chair's backrest two feet away from it.

2. From this position, straighten your arms and lean forward so that your hands are on the backrest.

3. Once you do this, lift your left leg backwards, keeping it straight. Ideally, you would have it parallel to the floor.

4. Aim to have your trunk parallel to the floor, and not only your leg.

5. Hold that position for a few seconds, then come back into the starting position and repeat on the other side.

Note:

This is an intermediate-advanced exercise that requires some level of coordination and balance. Before attempting this familiarize with easier variations.

Lateral Stepping

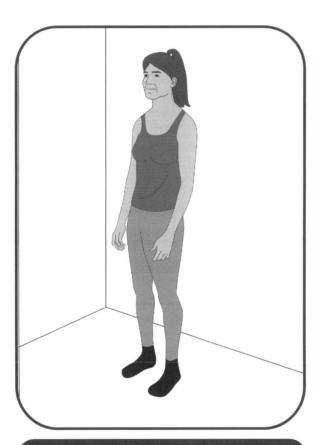

Step 1 - Stand

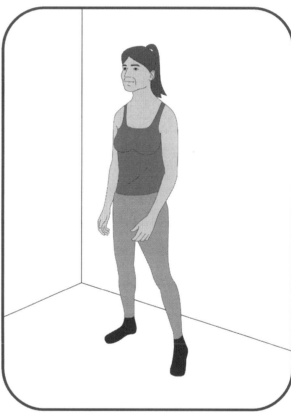

Step 2 - Take a small step on the side with no assistance.

How to Do it:

1. Stand tall with feet shoulder width apart and arms on your waist.

2. Walk with short steps laterally. Your leading foot just goes past your shoulder width in every step.

3. Perform 5 steps in one direction and then move to the other direction. This is one set.

4. Perform as many sets as designed in the program.

Note:

Quite an advanced exercise. Being able to move in a different direction rather than simply forward helps you increase balance, coordination and overall body awareness.

Foot Tap

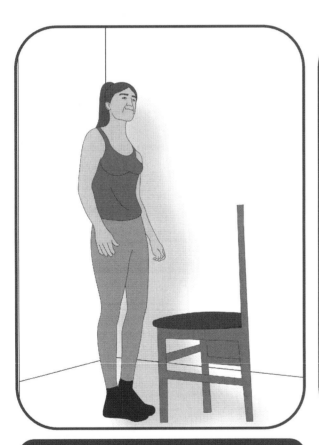

Step 1 - Startng position.

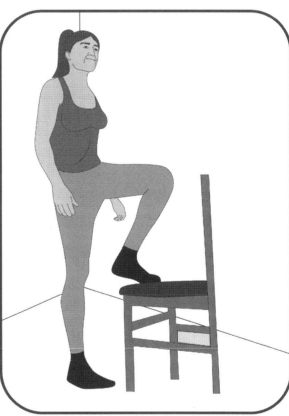

Step 2 -Tap the seat with one leg.
Then, repeat with the other leg.

How to Do it:

1. Stand in front of a chair two feet away from it.
2. Now lift one leg and tap on the seat with the sole of the foot.
3. Then, come back into the starting position, and repeat on the other side.
4. Repeat 5-10 times with each foot.

Note:

Very challenging exercise...If you can do this you will not only have the confidence to stand on one leg but also move freely in that position.

Tree Pose

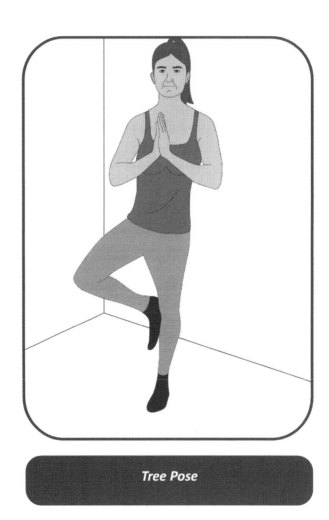

Tree Pose

How to Do it:

1. Stand tall with shoulders relaxed, chest up, feet hip width apart.

2. Raise your arms over your head and bring your hands together.

3. Then, lift one foot and place it against the inside of your shin.

4. Hold this position for either seconds, 10'' to 25'', or deep breaths, two to five.

5. Come back into the starting position and repeat with the other leg.

Note:

If you're coming from a period of inactivity or a surgery, avoid this exercise for now and perform the easier variation, Beginner Tree Pose Assisted (page.xx). Also, in this exercise it is especially important not to hold your breath but keep inhaling and exhaling softly through your nose if possible.

Three Way Hip Kick

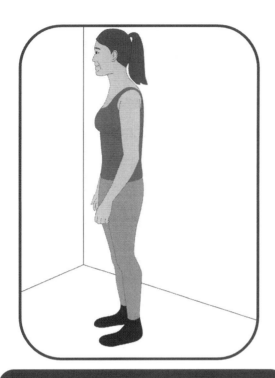

Step 1 - Starting position.

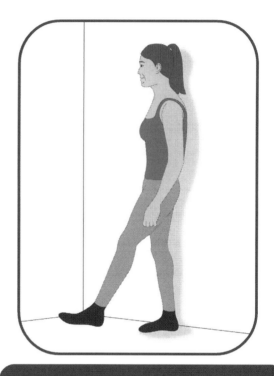

Step 2 - Bring your foot forward.

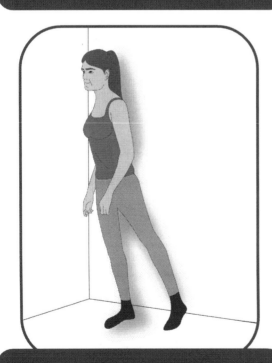

Step 3 - Then, lift is sideways.

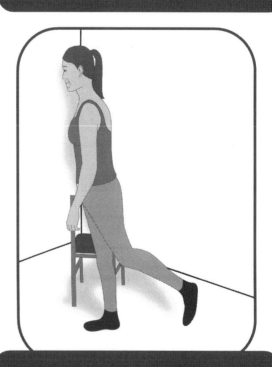

Step 4 - Then, lift it backward.

How to Do it:

1. Stand tall with chest up, feet hip width apart and arms on the side.

2. Lift slightly your left foot and swing it forward, keeping your leg straight. Hold it for 1''.

3. Come back into starting position, without letting your foot touch the floor, and then move it sideways. Hold it for 1''.

4. Once again, come back into the starting position and then move it backward keeping your leg straight. Hold it for 1''.

5. Repeat 3 to 5 reps and then switch sides.

Note:

This is an advanced exercise as you do not have any support to perform it. Great not only for balance and decrease the risk of falling, but also to improve hip mobility and foot strength, especially if done barefoot.

Single Leg Juggling

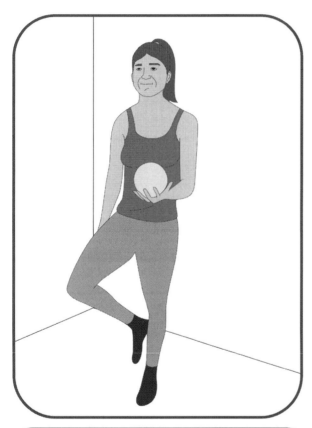

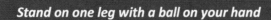

Stand on one leg with a ball on your hand

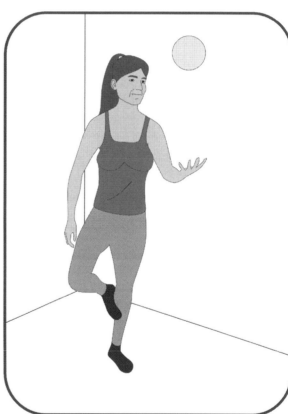

Throw it and catch it standind on one leg.

How to Do it:

1. Stand on your left leg with a chair on your right side.

2. Grab a small size ball with your left hand.

3. From there, throw the ball a few inches in the air and grab it again, still balancing on the left foot.

4. Do it 10-20 times and the switch side.

Note:

If you're coming from a period of inactivity or a surgery, avoid this exercise for now and perform the easier variation, Single Leg Chair Assisted Juggling (page.63). Also, in this exercise it is especially important not to hold your breath but keep inhaling and exhaling softly through your nose if possible.

Toe Touches One Legged

Note: I do not think you need this exercise to improve your balance and gain confidence when doing daily activities. However, If you have come this far, you might want to try the most advanced exercise available. Only 1% of seniors I have trained were able to do this. So, if you are among them, well done!

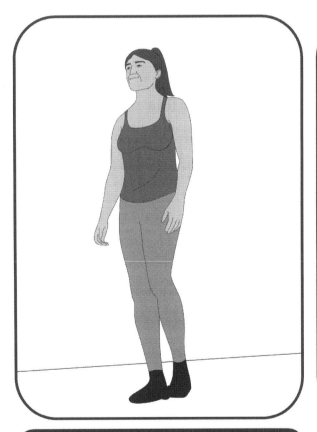

Stand on one leg.

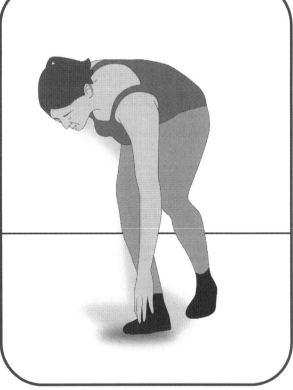

Touch your toes with your hand, whilst standing on one leg.

How to Do it:

1. Stand tall with shoulders relaxed and feet hip width apart or slightly closer.
2. Lift your left foot slightly off the floor.
3. Now squat down (or hinge at the hips) so that your left hand touches your right foot.
4. Come back into standing position and repeat on the other side.

Note:

Do this exercise only when all the previous ones have been mastered. One of the hardest exercises here! If you can master both sides, you will never have any problem of falling or losing balance. Guaranteed.

Some people prefer doing it squatting down, but this might put too much pressure on your knees.

Other people would prefer to do it hinging at the hips. However, this might put too much pressure on your low back.

For an extra challenge, try doing it whilst closing your eyes…. Definitely super advanced balance exercise, so be considerate.

4-WEEK WORKOUT ADVANCED PLAN

Congratulations, you have reached the last step!

Based on the amount of time you have and the energy level, you might perform these exercises for more sets.

For example, Day 1 includes three exercises. The minimum would be to do these four exercises for three sets.. However, you can perform it up to five times.

WEEK 1

DAY 1 - Perform 3 to 5 sets.

EXERCISE	SETS	PAGE
Single Leg T Shape	7 times for each leg	PAG. 75
Foot Tap	5 times for each foot	PAG. 81
Single Leg Juggling	10 times for each leg	PAG. 87

DAY 2 - Perform 3 to 5 sets.

EXERCISE	SETS	PAGE
Warrior Pose Hands on Backrest	5 reps on each side	PAG. 77
Tree Pose	2 sets of 10'' or 2 deep breaths for each leg	PAG. 83
Single Leg Juggling	10 times per each leg	PAG. 87

DAY 3 - Perform 3 to 5 sets.

EXERCISE	SETS	PAGE
Standing on One Leg	2 reps of 25'' each side	PAG. 43
Lateral Stepping	3 sets	PAG. 79
Three Way Hip Kick	3 reps for each leg	PAG. 85

WEEK 2

DAY 1 - Perform 3 to 5 sets.

EXERCISE	SETS	PAGE
Single Leg T Shape	8 times for each leg	PAG. 75
Foot Tap	7 times for each foot	PAG. 81
Single Leg Juggling	12 times per each leg	PAG. 87

DAY 2 - Perform 3 to 5 sets.

EXERCISE	SETS	PAGE
Warrior Pose Hands on Backrest	5 reps on each side	PAG. 77
Tree Pose	2 sets of 15'' or 3 deep breaths for each leg	PAG. 83
Single Leg Juggling	14 times per each leg	PAG. 87

DAY 3 - Perform 3 to 5 sets.

EXERCISE	SETS	PAGE
Standing on One Leg	2 reps of 30'' each side	PAG. 43
Lateral Stepping	4 sets	PAG. 79
Three Way Hip Kick	4 reps for each leg	PAG. 85

WEEK 3

DAY 1 - Perform 3 to 5 sets.

EXERCISE	SETS	PAGE
Single Leg T Shape	9 times for each leg	PAG. 75
Foot Tap	7 times for each foot	PAG. 81
Single Leg Juggling	14 times per each leg	PAG. 87
Toe Touches One Legged	ATTEMPT	PAG. 89

DAY 2 - Perform 3 to 5 sets.

EXERCISE	SETS	PAGE
Warrior Pose Hands on Backrest	5 reps on each side	PAG. 77
Tree Pose	2 sets of 20'' or 4 deep breaths for each leg	PAG. 83
Single Leg Juggling	16 times per each leg	PAG. 87
Toe Touches One Legged	ATTEMPT	PAG. 89

DAY 3 - Perform 3 to 5 sets.

EXERCISE	SETS	PAGE
Lateral Stepping	5 sets	PAG. 79
Three Way Hip Kick	6 reps for each leg	PAG. 85
Toe Touches One Legged	ATTEMPT	PAG. 89

WEEK 4

DAY 1 - Perform 3 to 5 sets.

EXERCISE	SETS	PAGE
Single Leg T Shape	10 times for each leg	PAG. 75
Foot Tap	9 times for each foot	PAG. 81
Single Leg Juggling	18 times per each leg	PAG. 87
Toe Touches One Legged	ATTEMPT	PAG. 89

DAY 2 - Perform 3 to 5 sets.

EXERCISE	SETS	PAGE
Warrior Pose Hands on Backrest	5 reps on each side	PAG. 77
Tree Pose	2 sets of 25'' or 5 deep breaths for each leg	PAG. 83
Single Leg Juggling	20 times per each leg	PAG. 87
Toe Touches One Legged	ATTEMPT	PAG. 89

DAY 3 - Perform 3 to 5 sets.

EXERCISE	SETS	PAGE
Lateral Stepping	6 sets	PAG. 79
Three Way Hip Kick	8 reps for each leg	PAG. 85
Toe Touches One Legged	ATTEMPT	PAG. 89

DAILY TIPS FOR PREVENT FALLING

Maintaining our balance becomes increasingly important as we age in order to stay independent and safe. Fortunately, there are numerous tips and strategies that you can use to prevent falls and improve your daily balance. In this article, we'll look at some of the most effective strategies for preventing falls at home, using assistive devices to improve balance, and making home safety modifications.

Preventing Falls at Home

Falls can occur anywhere, but they are most common at home. Luckily, you can take a variety of steps to reduce your risk of falling at home, such as:

• **Eliminating any potential hazards that could lead to a fall.**

 includes items such as stray rugs, clutter on the floor, and cords or wires running across the floor. Seniors can reduce their risk of falling at home by keeping floors clear and free of tripping hazards.

• **Improving lighting at home.**

This is another important step in preventing falls. Seniors should ensure that all areas of their home are well-lit, especially staircases, hallways, and other areas where falls are more likely to happen. Adding additional lighting, such as motion-sensor lights or nightlights, can also help reduce the risk of falling.

• **Using assistive devices to prevent falls and injuries.**

It can be beneficial for seniors who have difficulty maintaining their balance. Canes, walkers, and mobility scooters are among the many types of assistive devices available. These devices are great in assisting seniors in maintaining their balance while walking, lowering their risk of falling, and increasing their confidence and independence.

Other home safety modifications include installing non-slip mats in the shower and bathtub, using raised toilet seats, and ensuring that all furniture is stable and secure. You can reduce their risk of falling and maintain their independence and safety in their own homes by making these changes.

THE BEST FOODS TO EAT FOR IMPROVING YOUR BALANCE

I am sure are aware of the importance of having a balanced diet. Many studies and doctors talk about the importance of it to maintain a healthy lifestyle and improve overall well-being.

However, you probably did not know (until now) how some foods can improve your balance.

Here I am going to list x foods that will help you improve your coordination and enhance your balance while standing or walking.

- **Blueberries**

Other than having lots of advantages, such as being anti-oxidants and decreasing the likelihood of cardiovascular problems, eating blueberries helps with balance because of an ingredient found inside it called resveratrol which increases the brain and neural function associated to our equilibrium and balance. Recent studies have shown that blueberries have a huge impact on motor coordination as well as reducing "cell death" in our brain, making us feel sharper and less mentally fatigued...so make sure to get your daily dose of blueberries!

- **Cranberries and Red Grapes**

Like Blueberries, they also contain resveratrol and other small ingredients that will help with balance as well as longevity!

Obviously, they have lots of antioxidants (blueberries are still slightly superior though) and amazing for your overall health !

• Dark Chocolate

Dark chocolate is fantastic! Other than improving your mood and having some antioxidants, it is full of minerals that are often not present in our diets, making us more fragile, such as zinc, copper and manganese.

So, having the habit of eating one small (remember that quantity is important. Do not overeat it) dark chocolate would be fantastic for your health!

HEALTHY LIFESTYLE TIPS THAT WILL 10X YOUR FITNESS RESULTS

We are coming to the end of this guide...However, exercise is just a part of a healthy lifestyle, therefore I want to give you some guidelines to improve your health beyond exercise!

• Sunlight in the morning

This is an amazing habit that will change your life. Nowadays we spend too much time under artificial lights. Staying under the blue light all day is not good for our health and does not optimize our hormonal health. Even on cloudy days, going outside within an hour after getting up showed incredible benefits for overall well-being, focus and mood throughout the day.

In recent years many studies have been done on the importance and impact of sunlight, especially in the early morning as it helps falling asleep way faster, also improving quality of sleep, and releasing hormones.... Trust me, you would not want to miss these benefits!

For example:

• Mood and emotional well-being.

• Production of melatonin (released at night) for better sleep.

• Hormonal regulation.

• Ability to focus for longer.

• boosting and regulating immune function.

• Avoid blue lights before going to sleep

Sleep is extremely important for your well-being and fitness. Making sure that the quality of it is as high as possible is crucial (especially if you cannot sleep 8/9 hours at night).

Also, going to sleep at the same time every day will improve your hormonal health and make you more energized during the day.

Note: A general guideline to follow is to spend more time outside during the day and reduce screen time. Simple rule that gives amazing results in terms of health, productivity and well-being!

• Do not eat until you are full

It's not just about what you eat -however, try to include in your diet the foods suggested in the chapter "Best Foods to Improve your Balance" -; if you eat too much food, even if it is a natural non-processed one, you will feel tired. Ideally, you should aim to not go above 85% of fullness to avoid that feeling.

Also, drink more water throughout the day and prioritize good food that are minimally processed as it will be difficult to digest and most likely, not giving you the right macronutrients your body needs to perform at its best!

•Meditate 10 minutes a day

This is a practice that can be done anywhere. It might be easier if you find a slot during the day to keep it as a habit (as soon as you wake up or before going to sleep are very good options). You will definitely feel more centered, calm in stressful situations and in control of your actions if you stick with it for a few weeks.

If you have tried meditation, but you do not think it is very effective for you, try NSDR. It's a guided relaxation technique that helps tremendously! YouTube has a lot of videos about it that you can watch.

• Avoid alcohol

Many scientific studies proved that there are no benefits in alcohol consumption. A number of studies have shown that even modest consumption of alcohol can lead to increased stress and decreased resilience in the long run.

"Alcohol is the only drug where if you don't do it, people assume you have a problem." Cit. Chris Williamson

CONCLUSION

In conclusion, the journey towards balance for seniors is not an easy one, but with consistency and determination, it can be achieved. Risk of falling or not feeling confident in your own body should be something that you never have to experience again! I hope this book provided you with the necessary tools and exercises to achieve your goal of improving your balance and preventing falls. The division in three levels was meant to make it easier for you to assess what level you're at. In fact, if the exercises were mentioned without explaining the level of difficulty, I do believe it would have impacted the book's quality negatively.

Throughout the book, I have shared numerous exercises to improve balance through the exercises provided. For those who may be struggling with their balance, I want to guarantee that with these exercises, in just a matter of days you'll notice big changes.

I am sure that you will not only improve your physical health by following this routine but also improve your mental well-being. I understand that the exercises in this book may be challenging at first, but we encourage readers to stick with it. Consistency is the main ingredient of your fitness success, especially when it comes to improving balance. I can guarantee you that if you consistently practice the exercises provided in this book, you will see amazing progress in your balance.

I want to thank you for taking the time to read this book and for investing in your health and well-being. I hope that the information and exercises provided will help you achieve your goal of improving your balance and preventing falls. In closing, I would like to leave you with one final thought: regardless of your current circumstances, know that by doing the right action with good exercise, diet and sleep, your health will benefit and you will be grateful to yourself in six months.

REFERENCES

- *DeMark, L. et al. (2019) "Clinical application of backward walking training to improve walking function, balance, and fall-risk in acute stroke: A case series," Topics in Stroke Rehabilitation, 26(7), pp. 497–502.*

- *Dufek, J., et al. (2009) "EFFECTS OF BACKWARD WALKING ON BALANCE AND LOWER EXTREMITY WALKING KINEMATICS IN HEALTHY YOUNG AND OLDER ADULTS," Department of Kinesiology and Nutrition Sciences, 1.*

Made in the USA
Las Vegas, NV
15 January 2024